G000118209

Published by

British Mountaineering Council
Crawford House
Precinct Centre
Booth Street East
Manchester M13 9RZ

Telephone (061) 273 5835

INTRODUCTION

This short booklet aims firstly to outline the basic essentials of the *initial* treatment of an injured climber, and then in the second section look briefly at some of the common problems associated with expedition and high altitude mountaineering. It is not intended as a comprehensive textbook, but I hope those interested will be encouraged to delve further into the field which interests them most.

I hope you are not reading this sitting next to a casualty whose life may be ebbing away. First aid is like any other skill, you get competent at it by practising, and the more you practise the better you will get. There can surely be few things in life more traumatic that watching a close friend suffer or die while you stand there not knowing what to do. There are any number of courses run by organisations such as the St Johns Ambulance service, so get down there and learn how to give first aid properly.

The information contained here presumes little basic knowledge and the minimum of equipment. Although many things can be improvised, such as ripping up shirts for bandages, a basic first aid kit is always a useful thing to carry for anyone venturing into the great outdoors and the essentials are described in appendix 1.

Also included at the end is a short list of books for those who wish to read more about the subject.

THE BASICS

Theory:– Saving life is the priority. Worrying about spinal injuries will do no good if the victim is not breathing or has no heartbeat. The brain (which even the most dedicated rock jock possesses and needs) dies if deprived of oxygen for more than three minutes, so if someone is not breathing or has no circulation (oxygen is carried in the blood) this is the time limit within which you **must act.**

If there is a group of you around the victim and nobody seems to know more than you, take charge and issue instructions. Time is short and dithering may kill.

SAVING LIFE:– The easy way to remember this is **A.B.C.** – this stands for

AIRWAY

BREATHING

CIRCULATION

ACTION:–

The Airway:– being able to breathe is no good if the way in and out for the air is blocked. With your fingers, clear the back of the throat of blood, vomit, false teeth or anything else that may have been in the mouth at the moment of falling.

The commonest object to block the airway is the tongue which, in somebody unconscious and lying on their back, tends to sag to the back of the throat. (In somebody who is attempting to breathe, this will cause a choking noise.) Put your fingers behind the angle of the jaw on each side and pull it forward until air is going in and out without hindrance – *Fig. 1*. (If you possess a plastic airway this is the time to use it.)

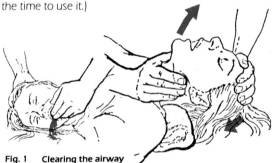

Fig. 1   Clearing the airway

In an unconscious casualty being transported, in whom this is a recurrent problem, a seemingly barbaric but effective way of sorting it out is to put a clean safety pin through the tip of the tongue, pull the tongue forward and attach it with a piece of string to the victim's belt or trousers.

Breathing:– I can tell you from personal experience that mouth to mouth resuscitation with someone who may have just vomited is extremely unpleasant but "A man (or woman)'s got to do . . .". To be done well this technique requires practice.

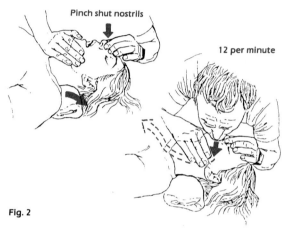

Pinch shut nostrils

12 per minute

Fig. 2

See *Fig. 2*. Tilt the patient's head back, pinch the nostrils shut (otherwise your breath goes straight back out, rather than into their lungs), take a breath, put your mouth over theirs and breathe out strongly. Watch the chest carefully. If it rises as you blow air in and falls as you let the air come out, you're doing it properly. You don't need to suck the air back out as the lungs contain elastic-like material and automatically deflate, like a balloon. You should be breathing into an adult about 12 times a minute. Don't stop until they start to breathe for themselves.

Circulation:– Do not waste time trying to find a pulse at the wrist or listening for a heartbeat. Feel for the pulse in the neck. Check it out on yourself *now* so you know where to feel if the need arises. If you can't feel a pulse in the neck (be warned – this may be weak in someone just having sustained an injury) start *immediate* cardiac massage. At the risk of being repetitive this needs practice to be done well.

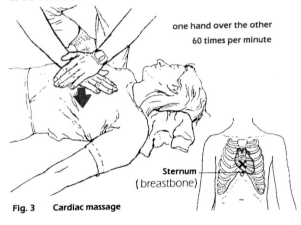

one hand over the other
60 times per minute

Sternum
(breastbone)

Fig. 3   **Cardiac massage**

See *Fig. 3*. Make sure the victim is flat on their back on a firm surface. Start by hitting them hard over the lower end of the breastbone. If this doesn't start the heart, place the heel of one hand over the lower end of the breastbone and the other hand over it. Using your weight, push sharply down, then relax. Repeat 60 times a minute in an adult. If someone is with you they can check that they can feel a pulse in the neck every time you press down.

If the heart has stopped, the breathing is likely to have stopped as well. This makes the whole thing a lot more difficult, especially if you are by yourself. If there are two of you, one can do the mouth to mouth and one the cardiac massage. Develop a rhythm of five quick compressions of the chest followed by one breath into the patient. You will need to change places intermittently as both procedures are tiring, but in different ways. Keep going:– people have been kept alive for many hours by this method.

If you are on your own, kneel by the head, facing the feet and develop the same rhythm, although this is obviously harder when you're soloing. Again from personal experience I can tell you it is possible to keep someone going like this for a long time.

After successfully resuscitating an accident victim, it is important that they are protected against further injury or the effects of cold and wet. For instance, in an area subject to repeated stonefall, the risks of moving the victim must be weighed against the hazards of staying put. It is also important for the person providing the first aid to be very careful not to fall or get injured themselves – more than doubling the problem.

Injured people are particularly susceptible to developing hypothermia and must be protected from the effects of lying on cold, damp ground and from wind and rain. (see page 29).

Having said all this, somebody who has had a severe enough injury to stop their heart and breathing stands a very slim chance of survival, even with the best of medical facilities. However, at least you have done what you can to even the odds, rather than stand by helplessly.

HEAD INJURY

Theory:– Due to the current trend for not wearing helmets, head injury of varying degrees of severity is regrettably becoming more common. In a recent survey of injury in Yosemite, not wearing a helmet was the single most common reason for preventable serious injury or death.

As mentioned earlier, the brain is vital, even to the most dedicated rock-athlete. A blow on the head from a falling rock, or tipping upside down in your harness and cracking the back of your skull, produces a disturbance in the level of consciousness ranging from a mild headache to coma or even death.

A severe blow to the head will produce injury to brain tissue. This is irreversible and any treatment is aimed at preventing further damage from such things as lack of oxygen or increased pressure inside the skull from bleeding.

Injuries to the spine in the neck are commonly associated with severe head injuries, so if someone is unconscious from a head injury, but is breathing and has a pulse, assume they have a neck injury and treat as outlined below.

Action:– Remember **A.B.C.** If the victim is unconscious, check they are breathing and have a pulse in the neck. Make sure the airway is clear and the tongue is not obstructing the back of the throat (see *Fig. 1*). Carefully immobilise the neck as described below. If airway obstruction is a problem or the victim starts to vomit, carefully roll them into the coma position *Fig. 4.*

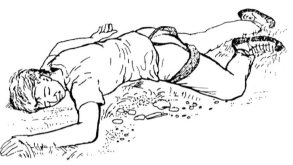

Fig. 4   The Coma Position

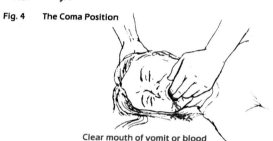

Clear mouth of vomit or blood

In mild cases the victim will regain consciousness fairly quickly. They are likely to be disorientated and confused and may be aggressive. Be calm, tell them where they are and what has happened, and reassure them that the situation is under control. You may need to repeat this many times.

The level of consciousness (how aware and alert they are) is the best way to judge progress and this goes from being alert and answering correctly about the time and place, through to being unrousable. If the conscious level is getting better i.e. more alert, all well and good. If the level is going down i.e. becoming more disorientated or unconscious – specialist help is needed quickly – evacuate as fast as possible to a hospital.

Do not leave an unconscious patient alone unless absolutely necessary. If it is essential, make sure they are in the coma position and breathing O.K. before leaving.

Anyone who has had a period of unconsciousness should be checked over at a hospital as it is possible to make an initial complete recovery and then deteriorate some time later.

SPINAL INJURIES

Theory:– The bones of the spine are stacked one on another stretching from the base of the skull to the bottom of your back. Running through them in a tunnel is the spinal cord – a bundle of nerves taking messages from your brain to the rest of your body. If subjected to a sufficient force the column of bones will break and move, damaging the spinal cord within them. This causes paralysis and numbness of varying degrees below the area damaged. Spinal cord damage occurs at the moment of injury and is usually irreversible. Only rarely does injury produce an unstable spine with little or no cord damage. It is this rare situation in which you can prevent accident becoming tragedy.

Action:– If somebody is conscious and complaining of pain in the back or neck, particularly if this is associated with 1) inability to move the arms or legs, 2) shooting pains down the arms or legs or 3) areas of numbness, decreased sensation or pins and needles – DO NOT MOVE, UNLESS TO SAVE LIFE OR UNDER MEDICAL SUPERVISION.

Neck Injuries:– In somebody complaining of pain in the neck or an unconscious victim due to a head injury, the neck needs to be kept as immobile as possible. A collar can be improvised from any stiffish material such as a magazine or just several rolled up pieces of material or from a double layer of cut up Karrimat (see *Fig. 5*). This can be passed carefully around the neck and tied at the front (be careful not to inhibit breathing). The patient should be flat on their back and the head and neck supported on either side to minimise movement. In hospital this is done with sandbags but you'll have to improvise – socks filled with sand or gravel, suitably sized bits of stone wrapped in material etc.

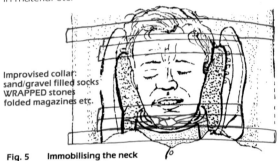

Improvised collar:
sand/gravel filled socks
WRAPPED stones
folded magazines etc.

Fig. 5   Immobilising the neck

Treat anyone who is unconscious or has had a head injury and is disorientated as though they have a neck injury.

Back Injuries:– Upper back injuries are usually splinted by the ribs unless severe, when paralysis of the legs will be present. Lower back injuries can be more unstable. If the victim is conscious and with it, allow them to move as they want. In the presence of a dangerous fracture of the spine they will be unable to do so. In this situation keep them as still as possible. If moving the victim is necessary to preserve life, transport on as rigid an improvised stretcher (see *Fig. 6*) as possible, to both prevent further damage and minimise pain.

Fig. 6   Improvised stretchers

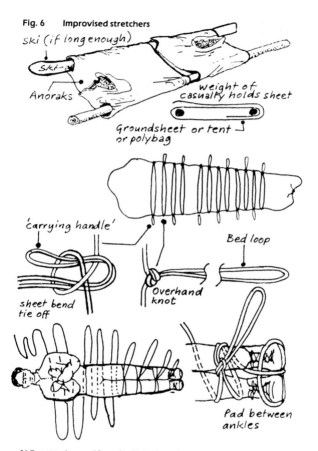

Ski (if long enough)

Ski

Anoraks

weight of casualty holds sheet

Groundsheet or tent or polybag

'carrying handle'

sheet bend tie off

Bed loop

Overhand knot

Pad between ankles

N.B. not to be used for spinal injuries unless there is no alternative

BLEEDING

A little blood goes a long way and makes many a strong man feel faint. Don't panic. Bleeding can always be controlled by direct pressure. If you possess a clean piece of material such as a handkerchief, fold this up and press into the wound aiming for where the blood seems to be oozing or spurting from (see *Fig. 7*). If you don't possess anything suitable, fingers will do. Keep up a firm pressure for as long as necessary. Elevate the affected limb – hold the arm up in the air or lie them down and lift up the foot. Tourniquets are to be avoided if at all possible, unless under medical supervision. Once control has been achieved, bandage the wad of material firmly to the wound (making sure that the bit beyond the wound still has some blood supply – press over the finger or toe nails and see if the colour returns. If you're really worried check the circulation in the uninjured limb and compare.)

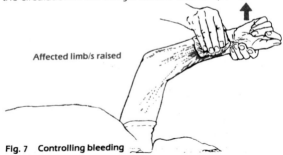

Affected limb/s raised

Fig. 7   Controlling bleeding

FRACTURES

Theory:– Bones are like pieces of wood. If you hit, bend or twist them hard enough, they crack, break or shatter – this is a fracture. The signs of a fracture are pain, swelling and bruising, deformity and, in severe cases, a grating noise as the broken ends rub together. A compound fracture is when the bone ends are exposed or have come through the skin. This predisposes to the complication of the fracture getting infected.

Generally speaking, there is no need to do anything to a fracture until reaching hospital except to stop it moving about. Movement of a fracture is VERY PAINFUL and tends to make people yell a lot – distressing for all concerned – so the crux of treatment is IMMOBILISE (see below).

If the bones are sticking out of the skin, just cover them with something clean and treat as above.

As always there is an exception to the rule. The deformity of the limb caused by a fracture may squeeze or kink a blood vessel, cutting off the circulation beyond the fracture. If the hand or foot is pink, and if you squeeze a finger or toe and the white area that appears returns to pink (compare with the other side), all well and good. If they are white to start with check the pulse at the wrist or behind the ankle bone on the inside of the foot in fractures of the thigh or shin – if they are present nothing needs to be done.

If there is no circulation, and medical help is likely to be more than a couple of hours arriving, the limb needs to be pulled straight. Warn the victim and be prepared for a lot of noise. Grasp the hand or foot and pull gently and steadily in the normal line of the limb, increasing the force until the arm or leg is straight. The circulation should usually return, so then proceed to immobilise. If the circulation doesn't return, it implies major injury that will usually require surgery – immobilise the limb anyway, in whatever position it's in, to stop pain.

Don't give the victim any food or drink, as when they arrive at hospital having anything in the stomach can delay the giving of an anaesthetic (often necessary for the treatment of fractures), keeping both doctors and *patient* waiting.

UPPER LIMB FRACTURES

ACTION:– INITIAL TREATMENT
Clavicle (collar bone):– Damage is usually obvious with pain and swelling.
Treatment:– a sling.

Shoulder:– This can be fractured or dislocated.
Treatment:– Don't try reducing a dislocation unless you know what you are doing and have the appropriate insurance. Support the arm in the most comfortable position. For a dislocation this will probably be away from the side, so put something between the arm and body. For a fracture support the arm in a sling and bandage the arm to the body to prevent movement. (See *Figs. 8 & 9*)

Humerus (upper arm bone):–
Treatment:– A sling or loop around the neck and wrist, and bandage to body.

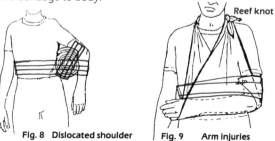

Fig. 8   Dislocated shoulder   **Fig. 9   Arm injuries**

Elbow:– Injuries to the elbow often involve the blood vessels of the arm as they cross the joint, so check the circulation in the hand carefully (see bleeding). If the circulation is absent and shows no sign of recovery after a few minutes, and you are several hours away from medical help, follow the procedure outlined above, but it is important to keep the joint bent slightly.

Treatment:– a sling in the most comfortable position.

Forearm and Wrist:– These fractures can be alarming to look at, with a large deformity.

Treatment:– As long as the circulation is satisfactory the fracture can be immobilised by lightly bandaging to a suitably shaped object, then rested in a sling. (*Fig. 10*)

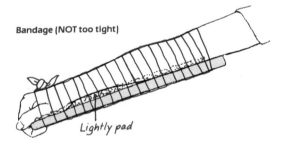

Bandage (NOT too tight)

Lightly pad

Fig. 10   Immobilising a fracture

The Hand:– These injuries swell quickly so keep the hand elevated by resting it on the opposite shoulder. Dislocations of individual finger joints are obvious and are easy to put back with a steady pull – *if you know what you are doing.*

Treatment:– Scrunch up some material into a bunch the size of a tennis ball and place in the palm of the hand. Lightly bandage the hand around this. Arrange a sling so the hand is resting on the opposite shoulder. (*Fig. 11*)

Individual injured fingers can be *lightly* taped to the neighbouring finger for support.

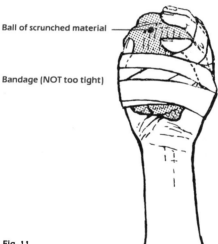

Ball of scrunched material

Bandage (NOT too tight)

Fig. 11

FRACTURES OF THE LOWER LIMB

These tend to be more dramatic as the victim is unable to walk, making the whole situation much more serious. The position of the Tibia (shin bone) just below the skin means compound injuries (where the bone ends are sticking out through the skin) are *a lot* more common and blood loss leading to haemorrhagic shock is also more likely.

Action:– Follow the general guidelines above. All lower limb injuries can be splinted by various means (*Fig. 12*) and usually supported by the other leg. Do not remove a boot for an ankle or foot fracture until in safe surroundings, as it will usually be providing excellent splintage. Once you take it off to assess the damage there will be so much swelling it will be impossible to get it back on again.

It is vital that fractures are splinted adequately before moving on improvised carries.

Fig. 12   Improvised splints   Do NOT remove boot/s (see text)

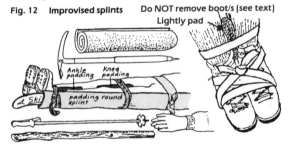

Improvised Carries: for one or two persons

Knowledge of how to improvise carrying someone with relatively minor injuries without recourse to outside assistance is invaluable.

It should be noted that 'one-man' carries are particularly exhausting! They are therefore of limited use for short distances only by the fit and strong. Even with a small group, carrying an injured person is still an exhausting exercise in negotiating what will always be difficult terrain.

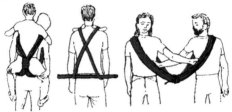

'Split rope'   Crossed slings   Double 'split rope'

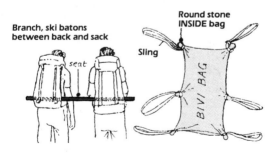

Branch, ski batons
between back and sack

seat

Round stone
INSIDE bag

Sling

BIVI BAG

MINOR INJURIES

Torn Muscles:– The sudden feeling of something "twanging" as you try to do just that bit too much is unmistakable. It hurts to move the affected muscle and it is tender over the affected area. Tears cause bleeding within the muscle and this causes further damage and delays healing. Treatment therefore, is aimed at reducing bleeding and is accomplished by Rest, Ice, Compression and Elevation.

Rest reduces further damage.

Ice cools down the tissues and minimises bleeding. Apply for periods of about 15 minutes intermittently, protecting the skin with a thin layer of damp cloth. Avoid this if you have impaired circulation.

Compression with firm strapping or elastic bandaging (be careful not to cut off the circulation beyond the strapping).

Elevation helps swelling drain back into the body by gravity.

Torn Ligaments:– Ligaments are the structures that stabilise the joints and are usually placed either side of them. A sudden sideways strain can stretch or tear them. Any joint that looks or feels "wobbly" after this type of injury needs a professional opinion. Rest the affected joint and support it with elasticated bandaging or strapping. Cool the affected area with ice (see above).

Tendon Injuries:– Tendons can be overloaded and snap. Extreme rock climbers put the finger tendons under enormous strains and can damage them. A sudden strain, as in trying to stop a fall, accompanied by a snapping noise and pain in a finger needs professional advice. If you have any doubts about whether a tendon injury is serious, seek professional advice. Rest the hand in a sling on the opposite shoulder in the meantime.

COMMON MEDICAL CONDITIONS

Many problems once exclusively the problem of the expedition mountaineer are now affecting the rock climber as our dreadful weather forces the dedicated rock star over the English Channel and into contact with nasty foreign germs and unusually strong sunshine.

DIARRHOEA

Almost inevitable in many parts of the world.

Cause:– nasty foreign germs or parasites

Prevention:– Avoid salads, uncooked food and untreated water. Make sure that food that has been cooked has been cooked thoroughly. Iodine based purifiers are best for treating water but taste disgusting. Once treated, water can be made palatable by straining through commercially available devices containing silver iodide.

Treatment:– Once it starts, avoid eating for 24 hours and sip plenty of fluids – treated water, still coke or black tea. At least with tea, you know it's been boiled. Electrolyte solutions, in packets, can be purchased at the chemist and are ideal for rehydration. They taste awful and are not really necessary unless you're losing a lot of fluid. When you recommence eating, start slowly and simply with small amounts of plain food. If you can get hold of live yoghurt it helps.

This settles 99% of cases in 24-36 hours. If there is no improvement or it's getting worse, or blood and slime appear mixed in with the diarrhoea, seek medical help – you've most probably got a parasite, salmonella or amoebic dysentry – this can only be sorted out by examination and culture of a stool specimen. In situations where no medical help is available, take Flagyl (only available on prescription in this country) or if this doesn't work, Septrin (also on prescription).

SUNBURN

Once the preserve of the high altitude mountaineer, but now often encountered in the peripatetic rockclimber.

Cause:– Too much exposure to the ultraviolet rays of the sun, (for those who haven't been abroad, that's the rarely seen yellow thing in the sky): particularly on sea cliffs where the ultra violet is reflected off the water, doubling the dose. At high altitude the atmosphere is much thinner and so provides much less protection.

Prevention:– Be very careful when first arriving in sunnier climes or high altitude and build up exposure to strong sunlight gradually. Invest in a strong sunscreen and smear it on liberally.

Treatment:– Calamine lotion for symptomatic relief.

SUNSTROKE (HEATSTROKE)

This is when the normal temperature regulating mechanism can't cope and the body overheats. The victim has a very high temperature, may be confused and delirious and their skin is often flushed and dry. This can be FATAL.

Cause:— Usually too much exercise in too hot a climate, coupled with an inadequate fluid intake. Humid conditions accelerate the effect by preventing sweat from evaporating.

Prevention:— Avoid prolonged periods of exertion in hot or humid climates. Stay in the shade as much as possible. Drink plenty of non alcohlic fluids.

Treatment:— Treatment is URGENT. Put the victim in the shade. Cover them with wet towels or similar, and fan vigorously. Encourage them to drink plenty of fluids.

INJURIES ASSOCIATED WITH COLD

SNOWBLINDNESS

Cause:– Excessive ultraviolet light causing a "burn" of the surface of the eyeball. This is commoner in the mountains because of the amount of light reflected off the snow. Symptoms often appear several hours after exposure and the eyes feel as though they are full of grit and become inflamed and swollen, causing temporary blindness.

Prevention:– Properly fitted snow goggles. If these are lost you'll have to improvise along the lines in *Fig. 13*.

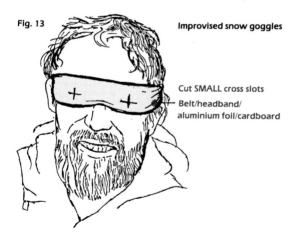

Fig. 13　　　　　　　**Improvised snow goggles**

Cut SMALL cross slots
Belt/headband/
aluminium foil/cardboard

Treatment:— Anaesthetic drops should only be used on a temporary basis to allow evacuation to basecamp. Bathing in cold water and the wearing of dark glasses can provide some relief. Infection should be treated with antibiotic drops.

HYPOTHERMIA

Theory:— As the body core cools, its functions gradually slow down and stop. This causes symptoms varying from mild confusion, incoordination and lethargy, to coma. A core temperature (measured rectally) below 32 degrees centigrade (normally 37) is very serious. Profound hypothermia, such as occurs in bodies trapped in snow for a prolonged period after avalanche, can put the body into a state of suspended animation, leading to difficulties in deciding when somebody is dead. People have been revived by specialist units, from temperatures previously thought incompatible with life. Don't decide somebody is dead until they are warm and dead.

Prevention:— Be adequately prepared for conditions you are likely to encounter. Don't forget that a large proportion of your body heat escapes from your head – "if you want to keep your feet warm, wear a hat!" and effective wind and waterproof clothing. It is important to maintain a reasonable food intake, particularly of high energy foods containing carbohydrate. In improvised shelters or a tent, adequate insulation from the ground is very important in preventing further deterioration from cold. If possible, avoid getting wet and seek or improvise shelter early if conditions are deteriorating, as exhaustion accelerates the effects of cold. If one member of a party develops exhaustion hypothermia, other members may soon develop the same – so take decisive action early rather than late.

Treatment:– If practical, remove wet clothing and replace with dry. Warm slowly. If the temperature is very low, rapid rewarming may cause fatal cardiac arrythmias. Wrapping in a space blanket inside a sleeping bag in warm surroundings is as good as anything if more elaborate facilities are not available. If trapped out in extreme conditions, get friendly and share your heat with the victim by sharing a bag. Hypothermia victims are often dehydrated and so if they are conscious, encourage fluids. If available, intravenous fluids are helpful when the victim is unconscious. To have the best outlook, profound hypothermia needs specialist treatment with intensive care and cardio-pulmonary by-pass facilities available.

COLD INJURY

Theory:– Because the body is largely composed of water, very cold temperatures cause localised freezing of vulnerable areas, usually the hands, feet and face. This is more likely to occur if the body core temperature is below normal. The damaged tissue behaves like a burn and is usually divided into two types. "Frostnip" where the freezing is superficial, and "frostbite" when the freezing is deep.

Prevention:– Adequate warm clothing. Avoid tight fitting gloves or boots. If practical take action before the freezing has become too serious and take time to warm up hands and feet as necessary. If with a partner keep an eye on his/her face for white patches of frostnip, which may develop without the victim being aware.

Action:– **Frostnip –** warm the affected area. Place your hand in your armpit or groin, wiggle your fingers and wave your arms about to improve the circulation. Feet can be warmed by placing in the armpits or on the body of a sympathetic and brave companion. Do not rub with snow. Be prepared for agony as the affected parts thaw out!

Frostbite – Much more serious, but initial appearances of black dead skin may be deceptive and recovery is often better than expected. If feet are affected it's probably better to walk down to safety on frozen feet and then thaw them out. Elevate the limb to help drain the inevitable swelling. Thaw the affected part in warm water (at 38 degrees centigrade) until affected tissue is soft and flushed red. Pain is usually severe during this procedure. Keep the area clean and dry. Infection can turn a salvageable situation into a life threatening one if wet gangrene develops. Avoid smoking (it constricts blood vessels) and give antibiotics. Spreading gangrene is the only indication for emergency amputation.

ACUTE MOUNTAIN SICKNESS (AMS)

(HIGH ALTITUDE PULMONARY OEDEMA/ HIGH ALTITUDE CEREBRAL OEDEMA)

Theory:– The higher you go the lower the amount of oxygen in the air becomes. This causes you to breathe deeper and faster to try and maintain an adequate level of oxygen in the blood. This affects the chemical make up of the blood and can lead to serious complications when the body can no longer compensate for the abnormal environment it finds itself in. Mild symptoms include headache, nausea, loss of appetite and breathlessness. The most dangerous complications are high altitude pulmonary oedema (HAPO) and high altitude cerebral oedema (HACO), which can KILL. In HAPO the lungs fill with fluid causing extreme breathlessness and in HACO the brain swells causing headache, confusion, lassitude, incoordination and unsteady walking, and eventually coma and death.

Cause:– The commonest cause is going too high too fast.

Prevention:– Acclimatise gradually. Once over 3500m try not to climb more than 350m a day. Spend a week at or around this altitude before spending a night at 5000m. If load carrying, go up and come back down the same day. There is some evidence that the best way to acclimatise for a big climb is to make several short trips to high altitude, returning to base camp each time, then make one big push for the top. Acetazolamide (Diamox) helps reduce the severity of symptoms and is useful for those prone to AMS. It does not give immunity to HACO or HAPO however, and does not allow you to go up to high altitude as fast as you like.

Treatment:– Mild AMS usually settles over a few days, providing you are able to rest. Severe AMS including HACO and HAPO requires URGENT action. DESCENT is the priority and HACO and HAPO can respond dramatically to a rapid decrease in altitude. Even 300-500m may help. Give oxygen if available. Drug treatment is secondary and only for situations where descent is impossible. It consists of powerful diuretics (which make you pass urine) to dry the victim out, and for HACO powerful steroids (Dexamathasone) to help shrink the brain down.

The use of barometric pressure bags into which the victim can be sealed and then pressurised, either by hand pump or with oxygen, may prove to be a significant advance in treatment if immediate descent is impossible.

After an attack of HACO or HAPO you should spend at least two weeks below 3500m. Recurrent HACO/HAPO is rare but can occur. If it does, you should think seriously about giving up going to high altitude – it's not just yourself you're putting at risk.

MISCELLANEOUS

BURNS

Theory:– High temperatures literally cook the tissues of the body. Burns can be superficial, involving only the surface, or deep (full thickness). Superficial burns do not destroy the nerves to the skin and so are very painful. Deep burns destroy all layers of the skin including the nerves, and are therefore insenstitive and painless. Full thickness burns tend to be hard and white, brown or black whereas superficial burns tend to be red. Superficial burns will heal themselves but full thickness burns will need skin grafting. Inhaling hot gases can cause burning of the lining of the lung – a very serious situation leading to difficulty breathing.

Cause:– Usually accidents with cooking stoves, or friction burns from ropes.

Prevention:– Be very careful with cooking stoves in confined spaces and letting ropes slide through bare hands.

Action:– Immediately cool the affected area with cool water, snow etc. for about 10 minutes. After cleaning, test the area with a sterile needle. If you can feel a pinprick the burn is superficial. Superficial burns should be kept clean and dry – cover with a non stick dressing. Full thickness burns will need specialist attention. Beware of infection in any sort of burn, and treat with antibiotics by mouth if infection is suspected. Initially keep clean and dry and dress the affected area as above. Large areas of burn leak a lot of fluid and protein and need very careful management.

ABDOMINAL PAIN

Theory:– There are a vast number of causes of abdominal pain, the commonest of which is constipation. The one everyone is worried about is appendicitis. Any abdominal pain that gets progressively more severe and associated with a high temperature and extreme abdominal tenderness needs a specialist opinion. Appendicitis starts with pain centred around the umbilicus which then moves to the lower right hand side of the abdomen. It may be associated with vomiting and/or diarrhoea.

Treatment:– Seek a medical opinion if possible. In the interim do not eat or drink as this will interfere with an anaesthetic, should this be necessary. If trapped out, in the presence of a temperature, take a combination of Ampicillin and Flagyl (two types of antibiotics – do not take any alcohol while taking these antibiotics) with the minimuim of fluid.

HEART ATTACK

Theory:– This is now one of the commonest causes of death in the British hills. A heart attack starts with severe chest pain located under the sternum which may also be felt in the left or both arms and up into the jaw. There may be sweating and vomiting.

Treatment:– The victim must rest. Ask about any medication they normally take for chest pain, and if they have tablets (usually "little white ones" for under the tongue) they take for an attack of pain, give them one. Send for help. If the heart stops strike them firmly over the breastbone, and if this does not restore the heartbeat (felt as a pulse in the neck), begin cardiac massage and mouth to mouth resuscitation as described at the beginning of this booklet.

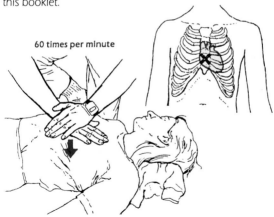

60 times per minute

BIBLIOGRAPHY

It is beyond the scope of this short booklet to cover all problems. For those wishing to read and learn further, I would recommend the following books.

Sports Injuries – A Self Help Guide by Vivian Grisogono publ John Murray.

Medical Handbook for Mountaineers by Peter Steele publ Constable (essential reading for anyone going on an expedition).

Mountaincraft and Leadership by Eric Langmuir publ Scottish Sports Council.

Practical First Aid by the British Red Cross Society.

Information on which vaccinations are required, and specific health problems of various areas is constantly changing. Up to date and good quality information can be obtained for a small fee from –

The Medical Advisory Service for Travellers Abroad (MASTA) Tel: 01-831 5333.

APPENDIX I

BASIC FIRST AID KIT

Assorted plasters

Triangular sling

Safety pins

Crepe bandage

Tweezers

A tubigrip elasticated bandage

A sterile wound dressing

Antiseptic wipes and cream

Steristrips (for holding wound edges together)

Zinc oxide tape

Paracetamol

All of these you can get from any good chemist.

In addition a plastic airway is very useful. This makes keeping the breathing passage open, in someone who is unconscious, immensely easier. You may have to get this from a friendly first aider or medic, and get them to show you how to use it.

If you are travelling outside Europe or the USA, it is wise to carry a supply of sterile needles, stitching material etc, as local supplies may be short and are often re-used without adequate sterilisation.

APPENDIX II

This appendix could help those who may find themselves involved in the helicopter evacuation of an injured person. Knowledge of the internationally agreed emergency rescue signals for helicopters and aircraft could help their crews effect a swifter and safer rescue.

The use of helicopters has saved many lives but they should generally be regarded as a last resort. Occasionally their use is essential to perhaps save the life of a person with very severe injuries and where it would otherwise be dangerous to move him, e.g. severe spinal injuries.

However, in remote country, high altitude and many areas of the world, their summoning and use often proves impossible. It should also be noted that although their crews are exceptionally skilful, they cannot fly into very narrow gullies, dense cloud, (usually) in darkness or exceptionally severe winds and weather, so consider the following.

DON'T BE FOOLHARDY

DON'T RELY ON HELICOPTER RESCUE AS A SAFETY NET

DON'T CALL OUT UNNECESSARILY

As an added word of warning, most countries, with the exception of Britain, usually charge either in part or in full for helicopter rescue and medical aftercare, so some form of insurance is prudent: it will save you severe financial headache, help avoid diplomatic incidents and could quite literally save your life.

The British Mountaining Council can offer sound advice on such matters.

That said, it is very useful to know the following International Code of Signals.

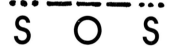

Whistle blasts or torch flashes (also large letters – see following pages for further signs)

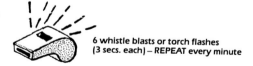

6 whistle blasts or torch flashes (3 secs. each) – REPEAT every minute

INTERNATIONAL SIGNALS FOR HELICOPTERS/AIRCRAFT

Signs can be fashioned from materials at hand, should be as brightly coloured/contrasty as possible and approximately 3m in size.

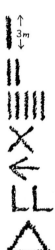

Require Doctor

Require medical supplies

Help required

Unable to proceed

Proceeding in direction of arrow

All well

Safe to land here
(PEG DOWN in centre of 20m × 20m) minimum landing area